Quit Smoking

My Way The Slow Way

P.J. Darnbrough

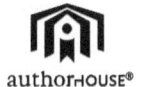

authorHOUSE®

AuthorHouse™ UK Ltd.
1663 Liberty Drive
Bloomington, IN 47403 USA
www.authorhouse.co.uk
Phone: 0800.197.4150

Published by AuthorHouse   04/17/2014

ISBN: 978-1-4969-7749-6 (sc)
ISBN: 978-1-4969-7758-8 (e)

A TICKET TO RIDE

When we arrived in Sydney Australia by Qantas in a Boeing 747 which ended up a turbulent free flight. I was allowed to stand in the cockpit for a few minutes and ask a few pertinent questions and it felt awesome, a great experience never to be forgotten. We were taken to a holding house in which we had to stay for three months. Problem was we had to be in by nine p. m. so this was proving a little ponderous to us so we decided that after Rob got a fulltime job we would move out and rent an apartment. As Rob was the only one of us to remember to bring all his documents with job references he ended up with a job first, on the buses as a conductor. We ended up in a townhouse in Paddington which was a two bedroom house. We were both nineteen years of age and we emigrated to Australia on a ten pound assisted package. For the first three weeks Rob looked after me financially paying for food, rent and cigarettes. I had only started smoking at the age of eighteen and it was also at the same time I had my first pint of bitter. I actually had a half of bitter with a bottle of brown ale which I mixed into the half. It was in the Elizabethan Hall at Belle Vue where the notorious Jimmy Savile was the resident D. J. Eventually I got a job as a conductor on the buses as well. At least it was a start for us and we were on our way on a new adventure.

Rob would go on to be a mental health nurse in Callan Park hospital and I would go on to join the Railways department in Darling Harbour as a clerk. I went on to do relief work after gaining internal qualifications which would enable me to work in booking offices and goods yards. It was good to be travelling all over New South Wales and ending up at places like for instance, Gunnedah, Tamworth, Burke and then back to Sydney where I was offered a new job in the posh Maquarie Street as an accounts clerk in a whole new set up that was computerised. I was earning good money and enjoyed the work for several years until after a separation with my first wife decided to get on with my life and move back to the UK. We had three children together and that made it very difficult to leave but I had to make a decision one way or the other as I was then very unhappy with life in general. So Manchester won my heart back, and I'm happy now and I feel I made the right decision for the time. The great thing is that I have a great relationship with my children still as we've kept in contact through all the years gone by. My family certainly helped me get through.

A WALK ON THE WILD SIDE

You have to have the right mentality to stop smoking. People who are weak willed or just plain whingers wouldn't stand a chance of quitting smoking. Most of those people are normally low in confidence and esteem. Show me a person who's glass is always half full and i'd tell you that that person would be capable of quitting smoking if they put their mind to it. I used to get them coming into the pub always complaining that life was against them and nothing in life was fair. Life is precious. I have actually talked some customers out of committing suicide by keeping them back at night and talking to them for hours advising them of the good things in life and to concentrate on them and not the negative side of life. You have a lot to live for and it's always good to always look on the bright side of life. One of my regulars was found in his bed by his mam who couldn't wake him and his father walked in an hour later and I had to tell him to get home fast and that he should take his friend with him as his wife had just rang with some very bad news. The sad thing was on that last night he ended up going to another pub before he took his own life, I think he did that on purpose as I would have talked him out of it. He was only 28 years old and I must admit when i'd finished my shift that day I went upstairs and told my wife and broke down crying.

To guide you through to the end, and quit smoking my way the slow way. Some of you might cheat and go straight to the end of the book and read the last pages and just read the method and how it works to quit smoking. But I would urge you to read the book from cover to cover and you will understand why you are stopping smoking and also learn how to keep off it.

Aesops fables tells us that the tortoise had a race with the hare. The hare was saying that he was faster than the tortoise and the hare ended up taking a rest and the tortoise overtook him and crossed the finishing line as the winner. The moral of this story is always walk before you can run. The slow way is the best way.

George Burns the American comedian lived to 100 years of age and smoked cigars for eighty of them. When smokers hear stories like that it gives them an excuse to carry on smoking, but let me tell you this, he was a one off, you don't hear a lot of stories like that because they don't normally happen. So no more excuses please, just get serious. Smokers who know why they smoke will find it easier to stay off the cigarettes when they finally quit smoking because they understand especially after reading this book why they started in the first place and understand why they are still smoking. They won't even feel the need for one cigarette or a celebration cigar for the birth of a baby because they won't feel like one or the need of one because they've achieved success the right way and are not suffering withdrawal pangs beause they've used my method to quit and it's pain free. When you start the plan, you will know from the beginning that when you finish my method, you will not be suffering with those nasty withdrawal pangs, because of the way you are doing it.

ADVANCE AUSTRALIA FAIR

When I was nineteen I made a huge decision to emigrate to Australia with a lad named Robert Evans who at the time was a boyfriend of my sister, who showed me a pamphlet depicting a few photos and sharing a few things that might prove helpful if we moved to oz. The main reason for me was the money, at the time wages on the average were $100 per week and I was on about 10 pounds a week, so in fairness it was an easy decision to make.

Australia taught me a lot especially in the field of earning money for a living instead of bludging it from the government in benefits system. In oz you have to work for a living, that is if you're an immigrant living in their Country, which I believe is fair. If you don't work you starve to death, simples.

Companies who make the nicorette patches are taking advantage of smokers who want to give up smoking as they are taking the proverbial "P". By using nicorette patches is really not the way to go to give up smoking or by using the nicorette gum or anything that has nicotine in them as it's simply swapping one addiction to the other, it's silly you should be working on a method for stopping smoking once and for all. Be serious. in life.

There's an old saying "Follow your heart, then your head, and then your gut instinct. By following that advice I certainly got myself out of trouble a few times, once when two lads spotted me and looked menacingly at me and as I was on my own in Stockport road, not far from where I lived I ran over to an older man, as I was only fourteen at the time and said to the bloke "Will you pretend to be my dad as those two thugs are after me"and he said yes and told the thugs to bugger off and they ran away with their tails between their legs. That's what I call thinking on your feet and following your gut instinct.

Always aim for the highest position in your job that you can achieve, chances are if you aim high and lose you'll be pretty far up the ladder anyway.

Practice your listening skills as an old saying goes, "Speech is silver, but silence is golden. We've all heard this common sense advice, we have two ears and one mouth for a good reason, so that we could listen twice as much as we speak.

Wake up, it's time to take control of your mind.

Self belief is one of the strongest allies to have. You have to believe in yourself to be successful at anything you go for.

You have to train your brain to think differently. Know that your conscious mind controls your subconscious mind and you can start to get somewhere.

ANY DREAM WILL DO

We all have dreams and we all want to succeed in life, it's in our D. N. A we all want to enjoy life, we all want to be healthy and stay that way, we all want to be successful, we all want money to spend, we all want to love someone and have them love you, we all want a decent job and we all want to lead a happy and contented life. I've mentioned before that I was shown both love and discipline. But sadly I've seen parents show a child their love but not discipline. They are afraid to dish out discipline because they think their child might not like them. So society ends up with a load of selfish people in the world who want everything for nothing. Lets hope that the parents wake up and start to improve our future generations. I noticed watching an old t. v. series called highway to heaven starring Michael Landon and Victor French, well in this particular episode Victor was trying to light a cigarette and "God" decided to shower him with lots of rain onto his head, it obviously spoilt the cigarette, so Victors character said to Michael's character "God must like me because he's looking after me. Wouldn't it be great if God could do that for us when we wanted to stop smoking. What a shame as we'll all have to help ourselves come off the dirty habit. The mind is a fantastic muscle, it's the source from which all perception, intuition, and movement originate. The state of our mind dictates everything that we do in life. All the great achievers of this world always had great strength of mind, and we're all capable. Also life feels better when you have a plan.

I believe that the fight against smoking cigarettes is similar to the fight against cancer as they both kill in the end, so I would consider the smoking of cigarettes is another silent killer which should be eradicated forever. It's just another killer that we've been suffering for years now. It's about time it was totally defeated once and for all. It's no good thinking back Well I shoulda, woulda, coulda!

A TASTE OF HONEY

Be confident in beating this addiction, you've got me on your side, and you have my method, and now you fully realize that your mind is going to take back control from your stomach. For years now your stomach has been dictating to you telling you what it wants to eat and drink. For instance if your stomach didn't like cottage cheese, your stomach would make you sick by rejecting the food and sending it back up into your mouth to vomit it out.

But if your mother made you drink milk of magnesia to settle your upset tummy and it tastes absolutely foul, you will still drink it. So in essence your mind is telling your stomach that the medicine is good for you and to keep it down. So your stomach is doing as it's told. So who's in charge of your body? ?

Of course it's your mind and now it's time to take back charge of your body and your destiny. Do it today and don't delay. Start quitting or begin a programme to stop now or soon. As long as you plan today to stop smoking sometime in the future. Your future is looking good already. So go for it now. You have me on your side. Treat me like your guardian angel and feel confident in your quest. Just think what your girlfriend might think or your partner of your breath, it is going to smell of a bad odour and it could kill the kissing so don't put your love life in danger. Think forward and plan for tomorrow to stop smoking and you won't regret it you'll only wonder why you didn't do it before. Wouldn't you prefer a taste of honey than a nicotine filled cigarette or even worse a bowl full of gunge from a smokers pipe?

BLOWIN' IN THE WIND

I think the government has worked out that the amount of money being used and wasted on the NHS by people who are smokers, drinkers, and people who are obese and overweight, far outweigh the taxation collected from the sale of cigarettes and alcohol. Thats why they've changed their tune.

They are building cars today whereby the driver has to blow into a device that registers a level of alcohol in your system and if you're over the limit, the car won't start up. Maybe sometime in the future they could do the same for the poor smoker and different types of drugs. The world is moving in that direction with it's new technology so it wouldn't surprise me.

Also I would like to see children being taught at school about the perils of smoking and provide them with all the necessary advice required to prepare them better for their future. Choices have to be made in life, do you want to be a decent member of society or do you want to be indecent and go the other way and end up a no-hoper and maybe end up a beach bum? If you're not going anywhere in life then you're going nowhere and it's about time you made up your mind.

You need to have an inner strength to beat your addiction and we all possess it, you just need to call on it every now and then to use it for your own benefit. Some people in life end up with many different kinds of addiction, smoking cannabis, injecting heroin, taking cocaine, sniffing glue, smoking cigarettes, cigars, pipes, being bulimic or anorexic, they're all forms of addiction and if we are to be free in life we have to liberate ourselves and it's o. k. to use other peoples help to achieve our goals. I'm going to help you with your addiction and we'll beat it together. Just follow my recommendations and you won't go far wrong. When you are off the drink and the smoking, then and only then does your body return to 100% fit, but also everything else that make up your system, your whole being, it's like having back the body of a fifteen year old that has never smoked or had a drink of alcohol. That is what you need to get back to staying fit.

BUSY HANDS

These days with mobile phones and computers and the internet and facebook and twitter everyone can keep busy with their hands as they're forever sending texts and playing games on their mobile phones. Also listening to their ipods. Some smokers worry about what they're going to do with their hands once they've stopped smoking. What do you do with idle hands? Well like I said before in todays era of modern technology you won't have to worry about that nowadays. One could also take up a hobby of maybe playing an instrument like a guitar or banjo or a ukulele. The ukulele and the banjo would be easier to play as they only have four strings to play on whereas the guitar comes with 6 or 12 strings. With all of these instruments you can learn to play with the help of the internet on youtube. You could watch George Formby play on the banjo and go on to learn the words to his songs and learn the different chords. He wrote some fabulous songs. Today we're all a lot more intelligent with the help of the internet and mobile phones with their helpful apps and also in our schools with better teachers coming through to improve the pupil of today with more modern technology. One of the best inventors in the modern era today was Steve Jobs of Apple corporation who invented so much of what we use today in our daily lives.

What happens to you in your life determines what type of character you're going to end up as either strong or weak. These are some of the things that happened to me to change my life forever. It was instilled into me by my Mother mostly during our childhood, but on one occasion my Father asked me to brew him a cup of tea. I was aged fifteen at the time and all I did was pour him a cup of tea from the teapot which had been on the stove stewing. My dad threw down the tea onto the floor and said"Make me a fresh brew, I didn't ask for stewed tea"He also added "If you're going to do something do it proper first time and you won't have to do it again"I learned a valuable lesson that day and got to appreciate my dad even more.

Life's not fair. Don't you just hate whingers in life. They're everywhere you go, everywhere you live and everywhere you work. They are always full of doom and gloom and carry the weight of the world on their shoulders. The old adage of the glass is half full or half empty springs to mind.

CHECKMATE

I used to play chess and took up the game in Australia and played many a game with the other lads that shared our house. There was four of us, Rob, Clive, Peter, and myself. We all played and built up to a reasonable standard. When I was working in Burke that is in the north west of New South Wales, I came into contact with a gentleman from Belguim who was a chess master. Well I must have played the lad about fifteen times and didn't stand a chance in beating him. What he was doing was covering all his pieces with other chess pieces so if I took one of his pieces he would always take one of mine He played as though he was a general in the army and I was a corporal. He was always planning ahead thinking 5 or 6 moves ahead. I would only think of my next move. Eventually I gained a well deserved draw which I was very proud of. He would have his pawns protected by the bishops and his bishops protected by his knights and his knights protected by his queen. Everywhere you looked he had all pieces covered and protected, just like an army. What I'm getting at is preparation and forward planning and then make the commitment and plan a start date. To plan is key. Feel confident about your plan and that you're going to win this battle.

But it did provide me with a great idea for packing up smoking and that was plan ahead and cover all angles and then attack with confidence and win the battle. By using a combination of self-hypnosis, will power, and slow withdrawal strategy I called it "Quit my way the slow way"and it worked for us. You must be serious about quitting otherwise you wouldn't be reading this book. So well done you've made your first step to quit. I'm determined to help you on your quest. It would also help if you are determined to quit smoking. Over the years i've tried many methods of stopping so now it's time to join a few different methods together and fight this battle head on together. It's a bit like playing a game of chess, start off with building a strong defence & base and work forward to reach your goal, and if you win it's checkmate!!

ELECTRONIC CIGARETTES

There are now E-cigs and also E-cigars and also E-pipes filled with loads of toxins in them. The W. H. O. are testing all the different toxins in the E-cigs and will be reporting the results in the future but at the moment, their thinking is that the toxins in the E-cigs are even worse than the regular cigarettes, and are causing more cancers in the human body. There is no tobacco in the E-cigs but there is nicotine so if you smoke these, you are still going to be addicted to them. Some Countries are trying to ban them outright. Even the very people who make these E-cigs have reservations about the use of them.

The big companies that are selling these E-cigs are saying that they are better than regular cigs and taste better as they have different flavours, including mint, and they are so much cleaner, ie, no ash, no tobacco.

The World Health Organisation have begun clinical trials and will be reporting to the Government in the future when they have the results. The E-cigs are made up of a battery, an element, and cartridge, and actually spews smoke when inhaled. The cartridges contain liquid mixed with nicotine. It' now called vaping and is big business. Generation 2&3 come with long life batteries. The government have decided not to allow these E-cigs to be advertised on television as a helping aid to stop smoking. Are they satisfying? ? To the smoker they may be, but if you are thinking of stopping smoking, I wouldn't recommend them as they wouldn't be a helping aid, it would be detrimental to you if you're thinking of giving up smoking. One person has been identified of dying from E-cigs as he was smoking 3o a day. They believe that the mixture of oil blended ammonia mixed with nicotine was the determaining factor that was found in his lungs. Three Countries have so far banned them including, Brazil, Uruguay and Singapore. Sadly E-cigs are being aggressively marketed at young children, and not a lot is being done about that.

All these companies that make the E-cigs etc, are hell bent on keeping you addicted to nicotine otherwise they're not going to make billions in profits. They will entice you with sexy and saucy advertisements to lure you into the trap. They don't care about your health or how long you live. All they're interested in is keeping you hooked and addicted to nicotine. They are not interested in helping you to come off regular cigarettes, they are only in it for the profit. Don't let them make you think any different. Remember the old saying Feed a cold and starve a fever. Well you should starve your system of nicotine, because once you take nicotine into your system, your system will always want more.

The electronic cigarette was introduced to the U:S: markets in 2007 and offered the nicotine addict an alternative to smoking tobacco. Most E-cigs are similar enough in to be mistaken for regular cigarettes, but one look inside and you'll see the main difference, E-cigs don't contain tobacco, instead there's a mechanism that heats up a liquid nicotine mixed with other chemicals which are poisonous and turns into a vapour that smokers inhale and then exhale called "Vaping"Manufacturers are saying that the E-cigs offer many advantages over the traditional cigarette but regulatory agencies and some health experts are not sure. They are all asking questions about the side effects of this new invention. Some experts are calling for them to be banned until proper research trials have been conducted to prove that they are safe.

The chemicals found in E –cigs are as follows:tar, the same substance used for road repairs, formaldahide, same chemical used to preserve humans, and animals, cyanide, lead, acetone, carbon monoxide, hydrazine, a chemical used for jet and rocket fuel. These chemicals are toxic and seriously bad for you and this planet of ours.

GREAT EXPECTATIONS

Your expectations are going to be enormous and very pleasurable when you eventually win the battle of a smokefree you. The success that you will create will form a new and vibrant future that you will come to love and appreciate. For the poor smoker, nobody likes him/her especially if they are eating a meal outside al fresco at a bar restaurant. There is many bar restaurants in Spain that are al fresco covered with an awning. That way the clientel can and actually do smoke regular cigarettes and is allowed by law in Spain. In the U. K. it is not lawful. It's becoming a sad world for the poor old smoker. The cigarettes are always going up in the chancellors budget and are becoming a bigger burden to the smoker. For a better pocket you need to stop smoking once and for all as the odds are stacking up against you and life is becoming unbearable.

To afford smoking today People are breaking the law by purchasing illegal cigarettes and also loose tobacco ie, golden Virginia, drum, etc, in public houses smoker and clubs. Roll-ups are worse for the smoker as they don't have filters with them, but you could buy them separate and put them in yourself. At least that might save the smoker mouth cancer if he uses filters. Do yourself a favour now and plan for your future, a future free of smoking to go and enjoy life while you can. You'll smell better for starters and if you're single and free, you will attract the opposite sex quicker and hopefully end up with an even better quality of partner, ie, a non-smoker.

HELP

In times of darkness we all need a beacon of light to come into our lives and that time has come for you. You have seen the light and now you're doing something about it. Well done to you for making the best decision of your life. Just think about it for awhile, you being a non-smoker, now make the most of it because you'll have more time on your hands, don't waste it, do something good and positive with all the new time that you will have created for yourself.

In my first year in Sydney i'd met quite a few people who for awhile became my friends, so we decided to venture out and seek employment in a place called Mount Isa where they had iron ore mines and there was the offer of a lot of jobs available. It's in the Northern Territory of Australia. So all three of us decided to thumb a lift and travel all the way by this method as we had very little money. We got a lift from Sydney and travelled up to the north of New South Wales and ended up in Surfers Paradise and went into a forest nearby. We settled down here for the night and I went off to collect some firewood and brush. Whilst I was in the middle of this a five foot black snake slithered just past my feet and I did not move a muscle I froze in that very spot. I was so terrified that when the snake went passed I sprinted back to the lads George and Tony and told them what had happened. They just burst out laughing. Then unbelievably on the same night a dingo walked into the camp and George went straight over to it and stroked it and it came across as very friendly. It definately surprised me as i'd heard they were wild and vicious and wern't to be trusted. This was turning out to be a great adventure. We eventually turned up in Brisbane where we knew an English lad who'd won a talent contest with a group by singing a song called "Little Bird"I spotted the biggest multi-coloured spider ever in my life and ran into the other room shouting to the lads to come and have a look. They were as shocked as much as me. The English lad named Alan said that there's loads. of them in Australia, they're everywhere. We decided to return to Sydney as our funds were running low. We didn't trust our luck to get any more lifts. So we travelled via Surfers Paradise again.

HERBIE RIDES AGAIN

Would you like to be healthier, potentially save a lot of money, have more energy, breathe easier and live a longer and happier life? Successfully quitting smoking can help you feel great, feel healthy, feel like a new person, and possibly save a small fortune.

There is a new thing on the market called SMOKE RX, it's a three step herbal and aromatherapy program that is supposed to be natural, safe and easy to use with no nicotine added and without drugs. Personally I wouldn't recommend using this as it's just another fad, why bother wasting more money on these silly cigs, get a grip and concentrate on creating a better life for yourself whereby you'll be back in control of your body and you won't be addicted to anything!!

Surely we all want that?

Ultimately you have to make the decision to quit smoking for good, no one else can make that decision for you. If you are not 100% committed to stop smoking, no product on this planet will help you. Please don't bother with these herbal cigarettes.

Also I wouldn't recommend quitting going "Cold turkey"as it's too cruel and bombastic and will hurt your body. Do you really want to hurt that wonderful body that you adore? ? NO! I should think not. Do it my way as it's pain free.

There's all sorts of different ways to quit smoking with the help of acupuncture, bio-resononce technology, home remedies, but again I would not like to recommend these as you're just wasting time and energy, why do it? Don't make yourself miserable, just follow my plan and be free from nicotine once and for all.

HIGH HOPES

Your health is the most imprtant thing to you in your lifetime and it should go without saying that it matters a great deal to you. You reach a point in your life when you have to make the big decision as to how do I come off the cigarettes and continue to stay off them for good, for the rest of your life.

It's going to be the most important decision ever in your life, so good luck to you for making up your mind to quit. The only thing you have to do now is read this book all the way through and plan ahead, and get started. There is now no doubt that you are going to quit smoking for good within the next six weeks. Enjoy the fact that you've made the right choice and go for it.

When my family moved from Dublin to Manchester in 1958 my dad collected us from the station and we arrived in Manchester in what was called a pea-souper, thick fog, it was as though we'd all smoked forty park drive in an hour, it was horrible, it was so bad we all had to hold hands and feel our way along the walls of the houses, and felt mightily relieved to reach our new house in Freme street, chorlton-on-Medlock.

To survive in life today you've really got to be on the ball, so if you're a smoker it will drag you down a slippery slope and it will have an impact on your workrate and you won't be as productive as the next person who is a non-smoker. The successful people who really get on in life are the go getters with loads of energy to lose and also people who don't have to whinge about how long they have to wait for the next break to have that damn cigarette. They are ruining your life so why not pack them in as soon as you can. Fred working in the next aisle is not waiting for a cigarette break, he's getting on with his work and he's probably doing more than you because your concentration is lacking because you're thinking about the next cigarette so you're probably suffering from withdrawal pangs. Non-smokers are usually more focused and positive and bosses love them because they get on with their work without the need to think about their next cigarette. These people probably have their own house or at least have a mortgage on it, also own their own car and go on holidays every year. Why is this so and you are stuck down in the doldrums with no direction in your life, no focus and no compulsion to get on in life, and no drive, sad but true. Do you really want to stay like that for ever? Or do you want to change the way you live now? Well now is the time to make that bold change of direction for the better, to make you a better person, one with determination and on a mission. Well I think you have realized that you were travelling down the wrong road and you have decided to wake up and smell the coffee beans.

I love my life now over here in Spain with my wife Linda. Because of the governments subsidy and the fact that my fiat 500 was twelve years old I decided to buy a new one from a Renault dealer called Martin Martin. I bought a new Renault clio That is beautiful and comfortable to drive. They have made fantastic advances with the technology in cars especially with the sat-navs. But the best thing for me right now is the fact I'm a non-smoker and have been for over two years and I'm loving it. I go out for a walk to the square to one of the bars for a coffee(cafe con leche doble) with my wife Linda. It's very friendly here with everyone greeting you with a hola or bueno tarde and with a smile. It's a beautiful little village in the mountains called Sierra de Yeguas, it means Mountain horse, Isuppose you could say we're living the dream. It helps being a pensioner now even though my wife's pension has been put on hold and she'll have to wait until she's 64, but grinning and bearing it as we're not the only ones having to wait. Back to the smoking. Some of you who decide to carry on with their smoking habit might be flatlining sooner than they think. It's worth thinking about because we all die at some stage eventually, it's just that normally we like to live as long as possible and we all strive to do so.

I HAVE A DREAM

Martin Luther King once said in his famous speech "I Have a dream". Well I have a dream by getting as many people as possible to quit smoking my way and become more healthy as a result. You are all being conned at the moment that you actually enjoy smoking and that it brings relief to you, but the sad thing is your subconscious and your stomach are being conned by a substance called nicotine which is a silent assassin, but you don't realize it yet it', s very cunning because it deceives you, it makes you think that you're enjoying it, but unbeknown to you, it's conning you, because it's very clever. It makes you addicted to the nicotine and just like the devil, when it's gets hold of you, it won't let you go. But also just like the devil when he's at his worst, you have to think positive. How you can help yourself reach your dream and stop smoking for good. It's positive and good if you believe, then you can accomplish something really good for yourself and improve your life, your health, and your bank account balance, and not be subservient to a drug called nicotine for the rest of your life. Suffering with anxiety is not a good feeling, and most smokers will feel this way at various times in their life and it's the cigarette that causes it, and it is the nicotine that's in the cigarette that causes the anxiety. It's not nice and you will have to get rid of it, and the only way to do that is to stop smoking. All the anxiety will leave you alone and you will be able to relax and enjoy life again like before you became a smoker.

IMAGINE

Can you imagine yourself to be a non-smoker in six weeks? Well you might as well because if you believe then you will. When you decide to embark on this journey, don't be afraid to enjoy smoking your last cigarettes, because it won't do you any harm no need to hate them. If you truly hated smoking then you wouldn't smoke, it's only because you're addicted to smoking that you are continuing to smoke, it's for no other reason. If smoking wasn't harmful at all we'd all be smoking and enjoying them. But because of what we've found out about them and the risk to your health most people are beginning to quit I don't blame them as it's the number one killer in the world today. Scientists have proven beyond all doubt that they pose the biggest threat to a persons life than anything else. They have proven that smoking does cause cancer to any of your organs fatty tissue in the arteries and veins, causes varicose veins and loss of limbs also basic deterioration of your body and health. The government of today are spending billions of pounds to get people off smoking and trying to promote good health, with the emphasis on more exercise and healthier eating habits. Cut down on the bad foods and eat more vegetables and fruit and healthy meats like chicken and pork and especially more fish, and less of the red meats like beef. When you've made up your mind to quit, go and enjoy your cigs and don't be miserable. You know why you have to stop and you're doing something positive about it. So don't be despondent you've made the right decision and you will go forward and enjoy your life.

You are giving up now because of what you know and also because it's the sensible thing to do. I don't regret taking up smoking in the first place, it was the thing to do in my day, and I was totally ignorant of the possible dangers attached to them. I even thought I enjoyed smoking them before learning all about the hazards. We've all been made aware of the dangers to smoking so we can't have any excuses to smoke now. I've just dealt with it and got on with life. I've finally learned the lesson. We've all made mistakes in life, it's how you deal with them and how you try and not make the same mistakes again.

IN MY LIFE

If I was a fortune teller i'd be able to tell you now that in a short space of time you are going to be a non-smoker but I'm not but I will tell you that you will be a non-smoker in roughly six weeks because you're Reading this book and you didn't buy it because you like to read novels, no it's because you are serious about giving up smoking, and good luck to you. The great thing is though you won't be needing any luck because you are going to follow my plan and use my method to quit smoking. I've introduced this method so you can give up smoking without any withdrawal pangs and anxiety, when a person quits smoking they have to go through withdrawal pangs which can be debilitating and cause you stress, so much that you might be tempted to light up again. But the great thing about this method is that you won't have to go through that pain barrier. Suffering withdrawal pangs is the one reason that smokers don't last the distance, with my method you'll breeze through it. Withdrawal pangs are horrible little niggly pains in the stomach and it will ache until you give it a dose of nicotine. You see at the moment your body needs a fix of nicotine probably every half an hour otherwise your stomach is going to remind you that you've not fed it with a cigarette so it's getting hungry for a cigarette otherwise the pangs set in to hurt you and remind your brain that you can't come off the cigs yet. Your body aches for a cigarette because it needs nicotine. The great thing is I've covered everything in my method so you won't suffer any withdrawal pangs. You will be able to come off the cigarette smoking slowly but surely.

Have you ever heard the expression "I'm in two minds"course you have, the sub-conscious mind doesn't think, but the conscious mind does. So the conscious mind is by far the stronger out of the two, ie, the boss!!The sub-conscious mind does all the absorbing of information and material and stores it for you in the memory box and lets your conscious do whatever it wants to. Normally the conscious mind will go through all the information stored and remove quite a bit to the recycle bin and file the rest for later. Sometimes just to annoy you it will deliver all the information to your conscious mind at the same time so you either have a meltdown or you end up with a massive headache, or at a time like bedtime when you can seriously do without the hassle. So the big thing here is to be able to relax and switch off so you can rest and sleep. You've got to be able to distinguish between the two minds and which way they work to get the best out of them. It's what makes you tick as a person. ie, your brains. Your personality and character are all formed by your brain, so its a good idea to know how it works. Use it to your advantage. Your conscious mind should be able to think clearly and without distraction for you to make the best use of it. You could liken your sub-conscious mind to Google on your computer. Google like your sub-conscious mind has all the information stored up in its database and you can bin any information that you don't need to the recycle bin.

My purpose in life is hopefully a life of purpose, Listen to your body, get feedback from it to know how to treat it best. Just by thinking and concentrating my mind I can actually lower my heartbeat. I've been able to do it since I took up Aikido. When after twenty three years of drinking alcoholI decided to come off it, my body would jump off the bed heading towards the ceiling because I was coming off the booze, it was like receiving an electrical shock, and I've had a few of them. It sent by body into shock. At first I was a little scared and I was beginning to think that it was not a good idea to come off it, but then I began to think of what i'd learned in Aikido and hey presto, it worked and i've been using it ever since. When my heart started to pump faster i'd concentrate my mind and bring my heart rate down and then i'd be able to sleep. My body would go into spasms, it felt as though I was going to have a heart attack, but after awhile i'd learned how to stabalize it. So eventually I was able to come off the booze successfully. It was amazing how much confidence learning a martial art gives you, I suppose I was lucky that the instructor came to the ymca that day to ask if he could hire a court big enough to train in and obviously we had. In the beginning the Sensi (instructor) hired the hall for one night a week and then added another night and then added a further day which was on a Sunday in the afternoon. I ended up spending a further two and a half years studying Aikido before taking on a new venture and that was buying our first pub in Dukinfield. Studying Aikido gave me a new confidence within myself to such an extent that I was never scared of handling people without fear. I was always able to stay relaxed and enjoy the days and nights without worry.

In the beginning

Over the years I have given up smoking four times. Once for ten months, twice for four years and lastly for one year. I have used different methods for stopping smoking and have been successful on every occasion except the first time whereby I had to persevere over a few weeks as I found it so hard to give up. But I kept at it and eventually was successful. My wife and I have been off the cigarettes for two years now and seriously would never contemplate going back to them ever again. I've had various reasons for quitting smoking and the first one was for saving money. The second reason was when my daughter came into this world and obviously wasn't going to endanger her health. The third time was to save up to buy our first pub. We had to give up the booze as well if we were going to be successful so we did it and went on to buy our first tenancy public house, which was in King street, Dukinfield, Cheshire. It was called the Newmarket Tavern It's in between Ashton and Hyde. We ended up staying there for fifteen happy years before we retired to Spain in November 2003.

Having just returned from a holiday in Australia where I met up with my children and friends, I couldn't help noticing that the airlines have even banned electronic cigarettes from being used. So it seems the whole world is changing and more and more people want to come off the cigs and try other forms of smoking to save money or to improve their health or even some other reasons.

Between my wife and I, we have four children, Katrina, Simon, Chris, &Barry. We also have ten lovely grandchildren.

When you look at the world now the poor smoker is being made to feel unwelcome everywhere, so the sooner you come off the weed the better you will feel.

You have to make up your mind before stopping smoking as if you're unsure it won't work. You have to be 100% committed before you take on the challenge.

You also have to make up your mind as to what is in control of your body, Your mind or your stomach? ?

If you are a smoker, it's your stomach that dictates what you put into your body. When you stop or quit smoking you'll be taking back charge of your body and your mind will be back in control as it should be.

Playing cards one night with my wife Linda, we were smokers at the time and without a car, so I phoned up a taxi company that we used quite often and got the taxi driver to pick up a packet of cigs for us and deliver them back to our house. It cost us at the time the cost of the cigs and one pound for the fare. That happens when you are well and truly addicted as we were. o. k. it was 3am in the morning but it's still no excuse is it? But sadly these things happen when your body is addicted to nicotine, which is the main ingredient in cigarettes along with thousands of other chemicals which are also bad for you.

When you are a smoker, your body is always telling you that you need a cigarette quick otherwise your body will go into shock, because your body is being starved of nicotine. When you feed your body with nicotine your body relaxes because it's had it's fix.

It's like being addicted to cocaine, a horrible thing and it's also the same for the poor old smoker.

All of our children don't smoke, and we are very glad, and because of that, more than likely their children won't smoke either.

The way forward is a three pronged approach, firstly forward planning, ie have a plan of action, a strategy, and secondly work out a start date, don't worry too much about a finish date as that will take care of itself, thirdly quit smoking my way the slow way.

I can't open the door for you, but I can give you the key.

Mark Twain once said, "It's easy to give up smoking, i've done it thousands of times. "

The reason for doing it slowly is this;Treat your body like a temple. They say obviously if you love your body, you're going to take care of it, and you don't want to hurt it one little bit. To stop smoking immediately is doing so without a plan of action, also if you've smoked your last cig, your stomach is going to crave a cigarette within half an hour.

You will suffer withdrawal symptoms very quickly and it does hurt. Your body is used to a daily dose of nicotine every hour or half an hour, and it's not going to be happy if you decide to starve it of nicotine without doing it very carefully and hopefully pain free. You've got to cherish this body of yours. By having inside information you will know how to be gentle to your body and take it nice and easy and slow.

The great thing about this method is you know you'll be off the cigs when you finish the plan, so no need to worry about a finish date. All told it will take about 45 days to complete. But the great thing is you don't have to worry about the last day, it'll just happen and job done. Say goodbye at last to that demon nicotine and goodbye for good. Hello life I'm ready for you now, time to dance, time to sing, time to enjoy the rest of your life.

I'm loving my life in Spain with my wife Linda. Linda loves reading novels that are fiction, and possesses great knowledge she has great stamina now because of quitting smoking two years ago, and also is now looking even younger. All my friends know I'm a musician and once I was asked if Linda played any instruments and I said "No" but she can blow her own trumpet! Sorry about that, couldn't help it.

We found it to be a lot easier to come off the cigs together as you come to rely on each other just in case one of you suffers a bad day. Luckily for us we didn't as I laid out the plan of action and followed it through to perfection.

We had bad weather in February but halfway through our plan I stipulated to Linda that all the cigs from now on we would have to smoke them outside of the house, and because it was in feb' it was absolutely freezing so it made smoking less enjoyable and more of a chore. At times it was perishing but worked out better in our favour.

It's a changing world. Do you want to be stuck in the doldrums as a smoker who can't or won't give up poisoning your system and suffer with the delusion that you actually enjoy smoking? ? Don't make me laugh. You've been duped into smoking by either your parents who smoked or by your peers/friends thinking it was a cool thing to do. Well today anyone who wants to know will tell you it's the worst thing that we could have taken up and all because of Sir Walter Raleigh, and all the big manufacturers. Those big companies with their advertising and clever slogans made it look so cool to smoke in the early days.

I remember way back in the 60's and watching an advert on the tv and seeing this bloke smoking a pall mall cigarette and looking pretty cool.

We were offered our first pub in town called the Rising Sun, on Queen street, just off deansgate, in Manchester. It was a pub that we had done a fortnights relief for the manager and we fell in love with the pub, so when we were offered it, we couldn't turn it down.

It was around the month of May 1981 when we took over after five months of training and doing relief work on the circuit. It was here that I got a good taste of the beer and enjoyed same. Being the manager I was being treated like a celebrity and enjoyed it immencely. Sometimes customers would offer to buy me a drink and I would accept. Also at times I would accept a drink at lunchtimes and found to my cost, that it made me tired and i'd have to sleep it off for an hour so I kicked that into touch, but I continued to drink at night, every night. I enjoyed the Carling lager at the time and would consume a few pints per night just to socialise with the customers and totally enjoyed doing this for the next 3 and a half years.

Sometimes I would start drinking at the monthly meetings that the managers had to attend as part of our contracts, and we would all get together after the meetings and go on a pub crawl and end up at one of their pubs. I personally enjoyed these too much for my liking as this was the only times when me and my wife would have a fallout. So eventually I had to curtail my drinking habits on meetings day.

If you are an alcoholic you will need professional help to come off it so you would need to book into a clinic.

But if you are just a social drinker you should be able to come off the drink quite easily. We come off the drink every year for a few months to regenerate all of our organs. When you drink alcohol every night without a break for a while, your body starts to lose the vitamin "C" levels from your body, so what I recommend to beer drinkers is when you are ready to come off the booze, go onto the hard stuff, have a couple of brandy doubles with orange juice and have a good sleep that night, and not drink the following day. The only thing that will happen is that you will lose a few hours on the first booze free night and even less the following night and then thats it. You are free from the booze . . . . and no harm done. Now you are ready to plan for your release from the addiction of nicotine.

I would recommend that you leave it for at least three months before taking up drinking again because you don't want to jeopardise all the good work you have done to come off the fags. Sadly when most drinkers partake in a beer/ lager they then need a fix of nicotine and have a cigarette. So don't do it and make it hard for yourself. Take things easy for awhile, and chill out.

We were ok to drink after coming off the cigs and waiting for a few months, so we went out on a quiet night and had a few drinks and we were not tempted at all to have a cigarette . . . . job done, no more worries whether we could or fail.

Well it's time to take back control and re-train your brain to take care of you and enjoy life without the added stresses. All you have to do is use self-hypnosis, and I will show you how to do it. It's very simple and no you don't have to be a hypnotist and it's certainly not at all dangerous. Iwouldn't show you if it was. It's just something I picked up a long time ago in Australia from a book on psychology. People of the world don't think it's possible to self hypnotise, but I beg to differ. It's very simple. It's just nobody has shown you how to do it. You probably don't know, but I'm going to show you now.

This is what you have to do:

Write yourself a brief note and start it like this:

I P. J. Darnbrough have decided to quit smoking in the near future because it's making me sick and I can't wait to come off smoking as it's stopping me from getting on with my life and enjoying it. This will take approximately 45 days

But I'm not in a rush as I know i'll be stopped within a period of six weeks because I'm using the method called "Quit smoking my way the slow way. "

Then sign it and date it from the time you start the programme.

What you have to do next is read the note to yourself twice a day, once in the morning when you get up out of bed, and then last thing at night when you go to bed. This you have to do for the next six weeks without fail. That is the self hypnosis programme, easy isn't it? ?

INDEPENDENCE DAY

Nicotine causes pleasant feelings and distracts the smoker from unpleasant feelings. This makes the smoker want to smoke again and again. Nicotine also acts as a depressant by interfering with the flow of information between nerve cells. Smokers tend to smoke more as the nerve system adapts to nicotine. This in turn increases the amount of nicotine in the smokers blood.

Independence day is your day for stopping smoking and you can start by choosing a date now.

Quotes and sayings are favourites of mine, especially the positive ones like; every cloud has a silver lining, and always look on the bright side of life.

It's always good to have a good outlook on life.

My parents had twelve children including one set of girl twins. My parents were called John and Bridget and their offspring the following names from the eldest down;Eileen, John, Marie Jim Tom, Paddy Tony Phyllis, Mandy, Sheila and betty, and lastly Ged.

At the moment the government are set to legislate against parents smoking in cars in front of their children. I agree with this as I think it's sad that the government have to make rules like this to protect children from the harmful effects from the smoke. Anothere thing the government are looking into is to stop advertising on the front of the packets, and end up with just plain covering.

If you are going to ever gamble, why don't you gamble on yourself. Forget the horses, bingo, fruit machines or playing cards. If you are trained in something like I was as a licensee in the pub game. I ended up backing myself to do it, So I gambled on me being good enough to achieve success in my own public house being my own boss. There's no better feeling in the world.

I knew of a chap who was a regular of our pub for awhile and he was a heavy gambler who would bet in the hundreds at times. Once he won over nineteen thousand pounds in one day and lost the lot within a week. So the gambler never gets anywhere because they're too greedy. They never have enough, how much is enough.

I also knew another lad who was a heavy gambler who at times won thousands and would you believe failed to pay his mortgage on his house after he won over 6'000 pounds lost his house after the building society foreclosed on him. What an idiot.

I did gamble on the horses for fun, and I never gambled more than a tenner ever because I used to gamble small to win big, and sometimes I would win and more times i'd lose but I ever only gambled with what I could afford to lose. That way you keep your betting in check and you don't end up in debt. The best way is for the small gambler like me is to put on your bet or bets and stay out of the bookies and check the paper for the race results the following day.

As I have learned the concepts in this book I have personally applied them to my own life and experimented and fine tuned my approach. I know from experience that they work. I was also after a simple approach to make mine work, that is why I came up with my method.

If you have the will, go and learn a skill and you will be quids in in the future.

I was born in Dublin on the 18th February 1948 in the year of the rat!At the age of ten I travelled with the rest of my family that had to stay in Eire for a few months whilst my dad saved up to pay for our fares to England wherby we ended up in Manchester. We had difficult times ahead in our schools interacting and making friends with other children as we were not liked by the English because of our accents but we soon realized that after a while when the other children got to know us for ourselves they pretty much took to us and all of us made friends. We made changes and the first was to learn the Mancunian accent and by doing so we were able to fit in better. I was signed up to join the Holy Name boys school and I got to love going as our main teacher was called Mr. Garside who was from Yorkshire and was a great teacher who taught us quite a few subjects such as the usual Reading arithmetic and Spelling, and Geography and History. He was a very fair man who could easily handle his class of forty two pupils and keep us all disciplined and well behaved. In the years that followed I ended up in the top ten at number six to be precise in all subjects and that's without the use of homework to help.

JUST STARTING OVER

I've made some big mistakes in my life and one of them was when we went on our first holiday from our pub called the Newmarket Tavern and booked a holiday to Albufeira, Portugal and we were really looking forward to it, and duly arrived in Faro airport and handed in our Passports to the desk at passport control only to find out that our passports were out of date by ten months, ouch!We were unceremoniously marched back onto the plane by four security guards who were carrying A. K. 47 kalishnokov rifles. They refused to listen to us and my plea to see the british embassy fell on deaf ears. I've never felt rage like it in my life but as it was my fault I calmed down and didn't put up any fuss, well I wasn't going to argue with security guards.

I made it up to Linda when upon our return to Manchester we then went down to London to renew our passports and then a new holiday to Gran Canaria for a fortnights holiday in the beautiful sunshine. My next big mistake was buying a timeshare apartment in Albufeira, Portugal for 3, 000 pounds, and ended up actually giving it back to the company that sold it to me. But I suppose we all learn by our mistakes and that's the main thing. It's not prevented me from going on and making a success of my life.

My Mother once asked me if she should continue smoking or give it up when she was 80 years old!My Mother at that time smoked about ten a day, so I or suggested that she carry on as is, because I thought at the time that it would cause her more damage and stress if she were to give them up. My mam went on to enjoy another two years. She lived in Northern Moor alone in a one bedroom house, and was a very proud woman. I remember when she was 80 years of age and she broke her ankle and she was asked to use a zimmer frame by one of the nurses at the hospital and my Mother said to the nurse"They're only for old people so I won't be needing one. "

My Mother was a wonderful Mother to all twelve of us and a great wife to my dad. Every road that you go down in life, you have to ask yourself is this the right road or have I taken a wrong turn metaphorically speaking. The main thing to learn is that smoking is bad for you and will eventually kill you if you don't stop.

MEMORIES

Quitting smoking can be a daunting task. Anyone who has ever tried it can attest to that. There were painful and physical and emotional withdrawal symptoms resulting the now absent and once comforting vice. Giving up smoking cigarettes is so difficult that about 90% of smokers who decide to quit eventually fail, but for every negative, temporary discomfort that a smoker goes through, there are permanent rewards for giving up the habit that can make the struggle worth it. Keeping these befefits in mind throughout the difficult process can make someone attempting to quit more likely to succeed, and eventually one of the many to succeed.

You will succeed with my method once you start it. It's really easy to go from start to finish and you won't suffer any withdrawal pangs using my method. Isn't that great news. When you quit smoking it's like putting a plug into that gap in your stomach that craves the nicotine from the cigarette, but if you ever start again by just having one, then you will be pulling back out the proverbial PLUG:Your body will start craving nicotine all over again, and within no time at all you will be back up to 4o a day!!

Within a few weeks of quitting and ridding your body of that disgusting nicotine You will be feeling great and on top of the world. You will be breathing better and you will also be getting out of bed with a hop in your step looking forward to the day.

Take one day at a time and keep a diary of where you are up to. Once you get down to smoking ten cigarettes per day the real fun begins. But you have to follow my advice implicitly and you won't go wrong. Stay positive all the way through and you will not fail. Don't despair if you fail the first time or second just start over again and you will succeed. Anyway you won't fail because I have confidence in you. The great thing is you are attacking this problem from all sides with a master plan so you can't fail. It's what all great football managers do every week to make sure that their team wins, and you are going to win. At least you've joined the right team at the right time and together we'll win this battle together.

MONEY MONEY MONEY

One should always strive to save money in a savings account in a bank, and this should be the money you have earned the hard way through working full time. It's more rewarding from hard graft than winning it at the races. Normally the money you win at the races is not looked after properly as you see it only as gambling money and not real money that you have worked hard for. You could liken it to monopoly money as you know you are going to gamble with it until you've lost the lot.

Lack of money is the root of all evil, said George Bernard Shaw.

Money is probably the most important thing on the planet, sadly, but we all need it to survive. We all have to eat food and drink water to survive and they're not free. They have to be paid for. You need a house, a car, clothes, everything has to be bought and paid for. That's why we're living in a commercial world. That's why we all work for a living to earn money and bring home the bacon.

We all have different reasons for stopping smoking but I will tell now that the top reason should be for your health, because if you are in good health, you have everything needed to get the rest. When you are in bad health you are constantly in pain, and suffer all sorts of problems like depression bad moods, or mood swings. The smoking stops you from doing things. Prevents you from walking, running, swimming, basically living a decent life. It's stopping you from buying a car. It's stopping you from buying a house. It's stopping you from thinking and seeing clearly all the pitfalls that you are fallng into because of your smoking. As the advert says on the packet" SMOKING KILLS" and you'd better believe it. It's the mother of all evils. Nicotine has caused more deaths in the world than anything else including mosquitoes. What more information do you need to convince yourself that what you are doing is seriously bad for you and will continue to be bad for you as long as you smoke.

NEVER SAY NEVER

Over the years I have given up smoking four times and most of the reasons why was to save money or pay off goods purchased on h. p. and also to buy a new car, and one other time I decided to work a full time job as a cleaner in one of the banks in Sydney as well as working full time with the railways department as a clerk. That was to pay off all debts incurred for buying goods on h. p and also to buy another car. I accomplished my goal in twelve months, and was very proud of myself as we had three small children by now. Katrina, Simon & Chris.

I moved to Australia in April 1967 on a 10 pounds assisted passage as they called it then. One of my sisters boyfriends named Robert Evans who lived on the opposite side of the road in Freme street, Chorlton-on-Medlock, Manchester. In England from the year after I left school in 1963 I started work as an apprentice engineer at A:E:I:metrovicks, in Trafford Park for two and a half years. Also worked for G:U:S:in Devonshire street as a credit sanction clerk for a further couple of years.

We were both accepted as immigrants to Australia and received a telegram within a week of being accepted. We had to go to a phone booth and call Australia house reverse call at a certain time. We were asked to make up our minds straight away to make a choice of travelling to Oz by aeroplane or go by boat which would take six weeks. The Qantas 'plane would take 24 hours, and we'd arrive in Sydney airport. We had to fly down to London from Manchester Ringway airport, and stay overnight in a decent hotel in Baker street(Sherlock Holmes territory)We were both smokers then.

Some people in Australia used to hire people to follow them and throw a pungent mixture of nicotine and left-over cigarettes mixed with other gunge over them to try and encourage them to stop smoking and also embarrass them into it in front of their friends. We won't have to go that far with my method, you can relax.

OH SO QUIET

Don't tell anyone that you're going to give up smoking, apart from your partner if you have one, but anyone else no! It will only add stress to yourself and end up putting a dampner on your goal. It's amazing when maybe down the line, somebody says something like, "Hey, how come you're not smoking anymore? " and you reply gleefully "I've given them up and havn't smoked in over three months, and what's more I don't even miss them!

Before tobacco came into our country, we would surely all be in better health and not be addicted to nicotine. I'ts only in the past thirty years that we've found out to our peril that smoking cigs and cigars are bad for you and cause cancer of various degrees in any parts of our bodies, but mainly in your lungs and throat, but also in your secondary organs, including the kidneys, liver, pancreas, stomach, and brains. It can also cause all these in our veins and arteries as smoking causes our blood to flow more slowly because our arteries are thickening with fatty tissue through the intake of nicotine which causes it.

When I think about it, I still can't believe that these big tobacco companies are still allowed to sell poisonous cigarettes to the public and get away with it. It's about time the government took up the case and put them out of business. We've all been duped all these years and they're getting away with it. It's time to put a stop to all of them once and for all. I was once asked a peculiar question"Would you rather face an Athiest with a gun, or a Christian with a gun". And I said"I'd prefer to not face either of them even though I was raised up as a Christian". That was a judgemental question, and shouldn't have been asked in the first place. We shouldn't be judged by others only by ourselves. Our opinions count for something.

RUBBER BALL

Your brain has to make up it's mind what foods you are going to eat and drink to keep your body fit and healthy. It also has to make up it's mind whether to allow poisons or toxins into your body. Strangely enough a lot of people including me had decided to smoke for relaxation purposes. That was a silly idea as it doesn't relax you, it just makes you more tense. It's got to the stage now that everyone is seeing smoking for what it is, and that it is a dirty and filthy habit that each and everyone of us has to fight and win the battle. But knowing that it is really bad for you, should make the battle to win that much easier.

Smoking in Spain where I live is still not being recognised as a bad habit overall as they're oblivious to the dangers. They're buryng their heads in the sand. It has been socially acceptable for a long time over here, but I believe that things might change now because the people are not allowed to smoke in bars and restaurants. The thing is most of the bars are having awnings built onto their bars and restaurants for the smokers. So the smoker doesn't have to worry about the police anymore.

Another thing that doesn't help over here is the price of a packet of cigs is very cheap, around about four euros per packet. Add to that the fact that the government don't charge any taxation on wine also makes that product very cheap. So it's a happy lot for the xpats who have retired here for the good life and to live the dream. My wife and I gave up the cigs last feb 2012 and have never regretted doing so. We will never take it up again as we both know the dangers therein. Life in retirement is all about enjoying oneself, but everything in moderation.

Everyone wants to make a difference in their lifetime.

Be yourself in this world-everyone else is taken.

If Al Pacino or Robert di Nero said to you, smoking is real bad for you and it will kill you if you don't give it up soon. Would you take notice from them, two of the best actors ever from the movies, I think I would, but they are not going to say that, we're going to have to do it together.

Your life is your own, you don't have to answer to anyone else. You make the decisions for yourself, nobody else has to do it, now that you are over 18 years of age. All the decisions you make now are binding, binding for yourself. Always try and make good decisions for yourself, and try and think forward.

FOR YOUR EYES ONLY

If you want to re-inforce the message it's a good idea to read the message whilst looking at yourself in the mirror!

Once I gave up smoking after I took up a martial art called Aikido, at the YMCA 125 club in Whalley Range. The reason for this was because a few years before I fell off my moped after drinking too much and ended up hurting my neck, so as a result of seeing the doctor, he put me on a drug called Diazipam which was an addictive drug which I found out to my cost when I wanted to come off them. So I decided to come off them proper and easily I cut down very slowly and finished using them within three months.

Because i'd taken up Aikido I came off the cigs as well and the booze and enjoyed practicing aikido for the next two and a half years. My neck came good and never suffered with it after that. Thank goodness!

When we took over the Newmarket Tavern on the 5th of July 1988 which is situated at 108 King street, Dukinfield, Cheshire.

After three weeks I started smoking again as I thought I deserved it after working so hard to get it. What an idiot

I was to do this as I became addicted to smoking again. I eventually went on to smoke golden Virginia Roll-ups for a long time.

We decided to quit smoking in February 2012. We both gave it up together. My wife Linda was smoking 40 tailor made cigarettes per day and I changed from roll-ups to tailor mades.

So I devised a plan of action to give them up once and for all. My plan was to develop a method that would allow us to give up slowly but surely so I came up with this metod that I call "Quit smoking my Way the Slow Way"

Because of what i've learned in the past and quit smoking using different methods, i've put three together to improve the chances of quitting.

SMOKE GETS IN YOUR EYES

One should seek good habits to keep and get rid of the bad ones, it will surely improve your lifestyle. We all strive for a better life don't we? From day one i've always wanted to be the best at what I did, from firstly the age of playing the piano at the age of six, a mere protoge. I would listen to songs on the radio and be able to play them on our piano which was situated in our parlour. The next best thing for me at the same age was football. I loved playing and from around the age of fifteen, I used to go to Old Trafford to watch Manchester United. I concentrated on mainly three players in particular, and they were Bobby Charlton, Denis Law, and George Best. I modelled myself on them and was fast becoming a decent player only to be stopped in my tracks when I was involved in a bad tackle which went wrong for me. Somehow my hip-joint sustained the injury from which I never recovered. Just as well I wasn't playing professional, as I would have been inconsolable, but I used to watch probably the best three players in the world at the time. It was an absolute privilege to watch them in action. Turning out to be a combination of the three of them would have been out of this world, Bobby for shooting, Denis for heading, and George for dribbling. I think God had other ideas for me. Enough about me. We are masters of our own destiny. Mark Twain once said"Quitting smoking is easy, I've done it a thousand times"Maybe you've tried it too. Why is quitting so hard for many people? It's because of the nicotine. Nicotine is a drug normally found in tobacco. It's as addictive as cocaine and heroin. Over time a person becomes physically and emotionally dependant on it. The physical side of the dependency causes unpleasant withdrawal symptoms when you try to stop.

The emotional and mental dependence (addiction)makes it hard to stay away from nicotine after you quit normally. Studies have shown that to quit and stay quit, smokers must deal with both the physical and mental dependence side of it. When you inhale smoke, nicotine is carried into your lungs. There it's quickly absorbed into the bloodstream and carried throughout the body. In fact when you do inhale the smoke from the cigarette which contains the lethal nicotine it reaches the brain faster than a speeding bullet. Nicotine affects many parts of the body, including your heart and blood vessels, arteries pancreas, bladder, stomach, kidneys, in other words absolutely everything and anything that is in your body will be affected by smoking cigarettes.

STORY OF MY LIFE

I ended up with a stiff hip joint as a result of contracting Tuberculosis as a kid I was about thirteen at the time and went on a trip to Yorkshire to a dairy farm whereby we were all invited to partake in a drink of milk from a milk urn. The milk was so fresh it was still warm. Unbeknowns to us was that the milk was contaminated with tuberculosis (TB) for short. As I was very fit at that time it didn't affect me until I was 17years old when playing football I was involved in a bad tackle in which my hip joint was damaged. I went to the doctor but had thought it might be a hamstring problem and said "Come back in a week and we'll have another look"After a week my leg felt alright so I didn't bother returning.

In Australia was the next time I had more problems with my leg, When I was getting up in the morning, my hip joint was locking and I didn't know what was wrong. A friend of ours who had an operation on both her hip-joints as she was suffering with osteoarthuritus. She advised me that I might have the same problem. So off to the doctor I went and after the tests came back positive for TB I then booked into the hospital in Tamworth, and had the operation. I ended up wearing a "Thomas Splint" for ten months and was confined to bed for the entire ten monthes. The staff at the hospital were quite brilliant and took me with the bed out for some sun quite often which was greatly appreciated. I was 24 at the time. As a result of the operation my left leg ended up one inch shorter than my right leg. It was 1972. The doctor who treated me and operated on me was called doctor Rowell and he said me that the inventor of the plastic hip-joint was from Manchester, England and was called John Charnley. The plastic hip-joint was made up of a stainless steel ball with an rod attached to fit into the top of the femur and plastic socket which fitted into your acetabulum. I believe that they've made more improvements to the invention and thereby making it last longer by using ceramic. I suppose that by having the problem of t. b. at the very young age of 24 years of age made me a very strong minded person.

When I returned to England in 1978 and went to the Manchester Royal Infirmary to see about a plastic hip joint. It's where the plastic hip-joint was invented. I was asked to come back at a future date and when I returned I got a bit of a shock as I was asked if 3o specialists could interview me about my request for a plastic hip replacement. I felt very privileged at the time. The main thing that arose out of the interview was the fact that I could sit properly and I could stand properly and also walk properly but with a slight limp. I was advised that the plastic hip joint would only last between 10 to 15 years only, so I was advised that if I was without pain that I should stay as I am and only think about a replacement in the future if I was suffering with pain.

You can't beat the power of positive thinking. Positive thinking gets rid of negativity in your thinking. and you will nearly always find an answer to any dilemma that you might encounter in your daily life.

SUBSTITUTES

Substitutes are a waste of time and money as you're replacing one addiction for another, especially nicotine replacement therapy, ie chewing gum nicorettes and nicotine patches and even the new electronic cigarettes with different flavours. What next? ? Only God knows. One of my brothers gave up smoking cigarettes 30 odd years ago and took up the nicorettes and is still chewing the nicorettes today.

Theres a saying: "The pen is mightier than the sword" but think about this one:

"The mind is mightier than the stomach"

The mind controls the whole body, make no mistake about that. You tell your stomach what it's having and sometimes your stomach will tell you it doesn't like something because it will make you sick and probably follow up by vomiting, so that tells the mind all the information required.

The mind will say to the stomach "Well your not eating that again as it made me ill the last time. But if you are addicted it's your stomach that tells you . . . . not your mind. When you are addicted to nicotine, it's your stomach telling you it cannot do without it.

Because of the addiction to nicotine, your stomach is telling your mind, " I can't do without this, it hurts too much.

So it's your stomach trying to tell you that you need to smoke a cigarette, and you allow your mind to be dictated to because the addiction is so strong. Well it's time to take back control and firstly "Train your Brain" to change your mindset and re-train your brain to think better.

I developed another method many years ago, a self-hypnosis method.

You write yourself a letter expressing a view to stop smoking by a certain date, ie, 30 days from now and write down the reasons for giving up, ie, it causes me bad breath, cost too much money. Make the reasons personal to you, that way it goes to a deeper rooted mind the subconscious mind, and read the letter every day, morning & night for the 30 days, will be re-inforced if read to yourself in the mirror.

I believe my new method is better because it's three pronged and covers more areas. It takes longer because it's better to prepare your body to accept what you are going to do. You're preparing your body with your mind through self-hypnosis and when the time comes, your body will not feel any stress and no withdrawal pains/pangs, because you have done it in a controlled way.

This definitely worked for me first time when I wrote the method, but I think this new method is better and stronger.

Always accentuate the positive, always think positive, be positive,

And stay positive. It's imperative that you do this, it's like the old song.

There's a spot in your stomach, the pit of your stomach which is the absolute centre point of your body. This is what gives a person balance. In martial arts it's known as your "KI"point where all energy can be generated, just below your belly button.

You're only smoking because you're appeasing your addiction, and your stomach is telling you that your body needs a fix!

Don't let your stomach dictate to your mind.

Live as long as you want, and never want as long as you live.

Be determined to complete the programme, that way you're giving it every chance to work, and it will work if you BELIEVE.

The big dictator

So we are going to let cigarettes dictate to us our whole life. I hope not as we all have a free choice as to what we do and what we eat and drink and also the choice of smoking or not smoking. I made the choice two years ago of quitting smoking and it's the best decision I have ever made.

Once you've made the decision to stop smoking, the rest is easy. It's just a matter of following the programme and at the end of it you're finished with smoking. The great thing is that you've chosen my book to read "Quit smoking my way the slow way".

Once you get started using my method you can look forward to being a non-smoker in basically 45 days, that's why it's the slow way.

You can look forward to your new life with renewed vigour and energy. You can begin to concentrate on all your other special talents to thrust you into a new lease of life and maybe try new things that you've been putting off. Because you've been bogged down with this addiction of nicotine. Now you can concentrate on new things and new beginnings. Be proud of yourself for making this brilliant decision to stop smoking. Now it's time to refresh that raw talent. Maybe you've played an instrument in the past and have neglected same, because your lungs were feeling weaker, so now that you're smokefree, you can take up the playing of an instrument again and enjoy life to the full. You can start living again and seek true happiness. We all have different ways of attaining true happiness. They say that true happiness is a state of being in perfect harmony with life, and we're all capable of achieving this wonderful feeling. You can do anything that you put your mind to, well that's what my Mother used to say. You can begin to be decisive again as you will be a non-smoker soon.

The humanologist

A punter will give themselves away by the way they walk as well as their faces. I would know whether they were drunk or sober within seconds of seeing them, or even any agressive behavior. The one's showing any aggression were always the ones to watch. Also one would have to look out for the underage. I once stopped a young lad at the bar and asked him for i. d. and he said he didn't have one, so I said well in that case you won't be served in here tonight, and he said "Who do you think you are bicycle face? Not very nice, but it did make me laugh afterwards. All in all, it was a great challenge and I loved every minute of it. They say that when you love your job, I t's not like work, it feels more like a hobby. I feel both privileged and proud to have been in the pub game for over 23 years. As someone once said, "If you want to knock down the wall between you and the life of your dreams, it's best to do it one brick at a time. I would love to inspire you to grow and be a good person and go on to achieve great things.

When I was working in Australia I did feel under pressure as the bosses were appalling with their manners. I wasn't used to being spoken to like that, like a Sergeant to a sub-ordinate. As a result I ended up working 16 different jobs in just twelve months, and I decided after that, that I would try and become my own boss, as I like to treat people with respect. It took me a while but when the chance came I jumped at it in July of 1988, and have never looked back.

I will probably be known as the last landlord of the Newmarket Tavern, as it changed hands in October of 2003, and was turned into flats or apartments by the new owner.

The secret to success is to be ready when the opportunities present themselves(Disraeli)

Now is that time and you have decided to come off the cigs, because this is your opportunity and it's not often these things happen in life.

THE LONG AND
WINDING ROAD

I'm hoping that my book will do it's job of helping people to quit smoking when they've made up their mind to quit and also be an interesting and enjoyable read. My wife Linda was taken into hospital for an operation on her stomach in 1993. She was supposed to undergo an operation for a partial hysterectomy but when the surgeon went in the operation turned into a radical hysterectomy. When the ovaries were sent away for analysis they were found to be cancerous. So Linda had to go on a chemotherapy programme wherby she was on a chemotherapy drip in which the liquid is delivered into the body over a two hour period in Christies hospital, probably the best cancer treating hospital in the whole of the United Kingdom. Linda in her first month of treatment was very sick as a result of the chemo. When we returned back to the hospital for the next bout of treatment I advised the doctor aboult Linda and how bad she was, he said we should have returned sooner. The problem was they always start the chemotherapy treatment with a diluted bag of the chemo' because it's cheaper so the doctor put Linda on the undiluted version of the liquid and as a result over the next month was a lot better. But Linda lost a lot of weight as a result of losing her appetite. She also lost her energy so stopped making the dinner. So that's when I came in handy and did the dinners for the next 18 months. Linda was to carry on with the programme for the next ten years, and was then given a clean bill of health. When Linda told me that she was diagnosed with ovarian cancer. We were shown into a private room where after telling me she broke down in tears. I said then we'll get through this as they're giving you the chemotherapy to treat this disease so just let that do its work and you stay positive and don't worry about the treatment, and we'll be alright together. I got through the T. B. and you will get through this scare. Linda ended up wearing a head scarf to hide the fact she lost all of her hair. That's when I decided to shave mine off and I shaved Linda's as well. Linda was on orovite for about two years which bode well for her as it was a multivitamin supplement which kept the colds and flu away. The main treatment was over a twelve months when she was treated with chemotherapy and therein after that with tablets and her blood was checked every month after that to make sure the medication was still working.

THE MAMAS & THE PAPAS

The sad thing about parents smoking is that more than likely, their children also carried on the tradition of smoking. It's also more likely that if the parents drank alcohol on a regular basis, then their offspring would do the same.

Well it's high time our generation got a grip and learned from our parents mistakes and not do the same as them. Also we have learned so much more about the damage that cigarettes contribute to the state of our health.

Our poor parents were basically duped into smoking by the big boys, the big manufacturers and by advertising and marketing strategies and ads shown on the t. v. and in cinemas. The film ad shown in the cinema would show a bloke smoking a pall mall and blowing smoke all over the place and look "cool".

The children of today are better educated and realize that smoking is bad for you, and now with the help of the government, there is no more cigarette smoking advertising allowed on t. v.

There is cigarette advertising being shown on the t. v. at the moment but what it is showing is the downside of smoking.

The latest advertisement shows a man inhaling smoke from a cig into his lungs and also shows the smoke sucked into the hearts valves and basically suffocating the lungs.

My mam and dad were both smokers, but my mother only took it up after all the children were born, all twelve of us. My mam was basically a housewife after her first child, but did work part-time at the midland hotel in Manchester. city centre, when the family needed extra money. My dad was a master bricklayer virtually most of his life, but was cut short when he fell off a ladder whilst working on a house on an estate and suffered a stroke as a result, but went on to live a further eleven years and passed away when he was 65 years old. I received a telegram from a policeman in Sydney, Australia, informing me of the death of my father, so I went over to my brother Tony and his girlfriend Jenny to tell them of the bad news. They were living in Coogee bay at the time in 1975.

My father smoked Park drive from a young age and although he cut down after his stroke continued to smoke because he enjoyed it. Sadly like a lot of people in the world thought they were good for you because they made you feel relaxed. They relieved stress when you were under it and they made you feel good when you smoked a cigarette, but the sad thing is they loved smoking for the wrong reasons. The thing is now we know so much more about the down side of smoking, we wonder why we took it up in the first place. In the early days nobody knew about all the chemicals especially nicotine content, but if people want to know about it now and all it's perils, all they have to do is look up the internet.

We had a customer in the Newmarket Tavern called Tony who introduced me to the pipe smoking club and lent me one from his collection, just a basic type. I was smoking roll-ups at the time without the filter tips which some people use to make the roll-up more healthy. Well I went out a bought some tobacco for a pipe from the corner shop and smoked the pipe for about three weeks. I gave it back to Tony after I broke my front tooth by biting down on the pipe. It did put me in a bad mood until I had my tooth fixed. Another regular called Eric had a huge collection of smokers pipes and they looked very impressive.

As every pipe smoker will tell you when you start to smoke the pipe and are at the infant stage of being one you will find out soon enough about the pitfalls, the main one being choking on the black gooey stuff that is obviously a mix of your spit and chemicals and the dreaded nicotine combined and is surely the worst ever taste in the world ever.

THE POWER OF BELIEF

What do we understand by the power of belief, well if you say, you keep on telling yourself that you are going to give up smoking over a few, weeks, eventually you will believe it. It's very similar to using self-hypnosis. What you are doing is re-training your subconscious mind to do what your conscious mind tells it.

Your subconscious mind is the bit that picks up all the information of the day and stores it for you to work on later. It'll store all the names and addresses of people who you have met in the day and stores it for you to peruse at your discretion. These days of mobile phones and computers with the internet, and facebook &twitter, everyone can keep busy with their hands as they're forever sending texts and playing games on their mobiles. They also listen to their i-pods. Some smokers worry about what they're going to do with their hands once they've stopped smoking. What do you do with idle hands? Well like I said in todays era of technology you won't have to worry about this problem. One could always take up playing an instrument like a guitar or a banjo or the Ukelele. The Ukelele and banjo are the easier instruments to learn, because they only have four strings instead of six that the guitar has, With four stringed instruments, it's easier to learn and you can get lots of help off the internet now. Also you can watch famous musicians like George Formby sing and play on his banjo. He was a great artist who wrote a lot of wonderful songs. Today we are all a lot more intelligent because of the internet and mobile phones and also in our schools the teachers that are coming through are more smarter than their counterparts and are teaching better because of new technology and techniques. The main man at Apple corp who died not long ago has made fantastic inroads with his inventions and we are all a lot better off because of him. Steve Jobs was the man who has enhanced our lives substantially.

I consider myself to be a humanologist a student of human behaviour. In my days as a landlord of a public house, my talent as a humanologist came in handy as when some punters entered our establishment, I would watch them like a Hawk and study their behaviour by watching their eyes and faces especially. I could tell within seconds whether I would serve them or not, and if I did decide to serve them, I would then consider whether to keep an eye on them or not.

As we all know you can end up with dangerous people coming into establishments wanting a drink and you have to be able to read customers to stay safe. The ones who are drunk are the worst ones as they can be very aggressive and can and do cause fights so the best thing you can do is just refuse them at the bar and ask very politely for them to leave and try somewhere else. I've never had a problem with a customer after I've asked them to leave and you've not only done yourself a favour but also the other customers that are already in having drinks and enjoying them in a quiet and friendly atmosphere. I believe it's the publicans responsibility to keep not only his staff safe but also his customers. Not all landlords believe this unwritten rule but I do. Over the years I've had death threats and also threats of violence and also just some insults but nobody has ever followed through with their threats and I'm glad of it, but it's part and parcel in our game. You have to get used to it and grin and bear it to survive. It's all about how you feel and treat it like water off a ducks back. On some occasions I've had to call the police when i've thought it may become dangerously out hand and they have always come out and got me out of a jam for which I was greatful. The police were always brilliant with me and said they were there at any time for us and to call them if needed. Luckilly over the years I've not had to use them too many times and we've always run a good pub and kept the idiots out. They only spoil it for the regulars and the regular punters will only take so much flack and will go elsewhere if you are not doing your job properly. Most landlords take their jobs seriously and have high standards and keep to them. Also I believe most of them do a good job.

THE PRICE IS RIGHT

I suppose the government is helping now by increasing the price of a packet of cigarettes. The cost of a packet of Benson & Hedges is 9. 75 pounds so anyone smoking two packs a day will be paying 19. 50 a day, & over the week a total of 136. 50pounds. That's over 7, 000 pounds a year.

How many holidays could anyone have with that? I'd say quite a few, and what about the car, does it need any repairs, or do you even need a new car, I think 7, ooo pounds would go long way towards a holiday or a car. Lets face it today cars end up being very expensive, with the m. o. t. to take care of and add the car tax, then the insurance, then the petrol, and just to annoy us more you have the poor youngster who is only in his twenties, he ends up being hammered by the insurance companies. Our Sam pays over 3, ooo pounds a year because he's under 25.

So the incentive is plain and clear for anyone who wants to quit smoking.

My parents sadly were brainwashed into thinking that smoking was good for you as they smoked Park Drive and seemed to enjoy them as they relieved stress and made you feel happier than before you smoked the cigarette. I am now

66, so it was a long time ago and our parents didn't know about the toxins and the chemicals especially the nicotine. But now your parents will know all of these things and hopefully pass on the good advice to never smoke a cig in your lifetime, and also explain why. It's only now that we know everything there is to know about the perils and dangers of smoking that first cigarette, because if you do you become hooked because of the nicotine which is probably the most addictive drug on the planet at the moment. It's probably as dangerous as cocaine, so beware and don't touch it if you can.

GENTLE ON MY MIND

The longer you smoke, the more you'll smoke and you probably won't stop 'till you reach 40 cigs a day. It's normally at this point your body says to you that's enough, "I've reached my tolerance level and I'm quite satisfied with that amount.

The same normally happens to drinkers, ie the longer they drink alcohol, the more they need to satisfy themselves. Normally with an alcohol drinker, they drink for many reasons, the main one being, they want to be merry and happy and have a good time. Depending on what mood you are in, the alcohol will exacerbate the mood of what you were in at the beginning, so if you were in a bad mood, chances are you will end up in an even worse mood.

Drinking and smoking are directly linked because in days gone by, it was the drinkers who smoked who kept our pubs going and kept us in business. The no smoking ban has doomed pubs to the graveyard.

Yes we had a smoky atmosphere in our lounge at the Newmarket Tavern, Dukinfield, especially in the early days, but a large ceiling fan that we had installed with the aid of an extractor fan over the side door put paid to the smoke.

Our first pub the Rising Sun had a resident ghost who was a monk who used to flip over ashtrays and beer mats when Linda was the cleaning in the lounge. On checking this out at the library, it turns out that many years before there was a monastery on one side of our pub and a nunnery on the other side, and one night I saw the monk who Linda called George glide from one side of the pub to go through the wall on the nuns side. I witnessed one other ghost in one of our relief pubs called the Fiddlers Three in Runcorn, and again he was a monk who was a poltergeist who threw around crisp boxes and ashtrays. What have they got against smokers? ? I believe the Fiddlers Three pub was built on sacred grounds.

Why can some people see ghosts when others can't? Well my answer is one has to be psychic to see ghosts because I can see them and my wife who is not psychic can't see them. It's the only rational answer I can think of.

Sir Walter Raleigh first brought in tobacco into the United Kingdom all those years ago and we've been paying the price ever since, but I suppose we have to be grateful that he also brought in the potato.

Sometimes you have to treat your stomach like a little child. What your stomach wants sometimes is bad for your body, but your stomach doesn't know any better, so the mind has to take control, because that's the thing that has the brain cells.

Going back to the ghost at the Rising Sun called George. My wife Linda who never saw him would shout out to him to stop messing about while she was doing the cleaning and he would!!

Over time the smoker develops a tolerance to nicotine. Tolerance means it takes more nicotine to get the same effect that the smoker used to get from smaller amounts. This normally leads to an increase in the amount of cigarettes required to fulfil the addiction. At a certain point in the smokers life he/she will reach a level that will satisfy the smoker and that level is normally reached at 40 a day My wife Linda reached 40 and stayed on that amount for the next 10 years.

When a person finishes a cigarette the nicotine level starts to drop, going lower and lower. The pleasant and fulfilling feelings wear off and the smoker noticeably wants a smoke. If smoking is postponed for awhile the smoker will start to feel miserable and irritable and start to get withdrawal pangs. Once these fellings start in the stomach the smoker has to have a cig quickly otherwise stress sets in.

The great thing is we have the weapon to destroy this bad habit once and for all, and it's called "Quit my way the slow way"and eventually I will show you the breakdown of cigarettes that you have to go through to win the battle.

At the moment it's important to know why we started smoking in the first place to understand where we went wrong and that way it's easier to fix.

Nobody wants to smoke really, it's because we've started and don't know how to come off them without hurting ourselves that we continue to smoke. I bet all smokers if they could go back in time and know the consequences we would definitely not take up smoking.

WINE DRINKER ME

To begin with if you are a drinker, you will need to come off the booze if you're going to be successful in your bid to quit smoking, otherwise you're just going to make it very difficult indeed or even impossible. So do yourself a favour and focus your mind on quiting the booze for about three months. If you are a regular drinker and basically drink to be sociable it will be relatively easy to come off the booze for awhile. If on the other hand you are an alcholic, go and book into a clinic because I can't help you. You will need professional help.

If you are a beer drinker change over to drinking shorts. Pick your favourite if you have one and have two doubles with a fruit juice and go to bed, at least you will enjoy a decent nights sleep, because the following night you won't have any booze, and you might lose a few hours sleep, and on the next night you might lose an hour, but that's all. You should sleep soundly after that and after a week you can start your new programme whereby you begin to "Quit smoking my way the slow way"

You might not think it will work, but it does. Make sure there is no drink left in the house when you drink you last doubles of spirit. Adding the fruit juice ensures that you body will retain it's vitamin "C"levels, because drinking alcohol reduces your levels of vitamin "C". By having the doubles, all you're doing is preparing your body for a calm and relaxed sleep. If you don't drink every day you shouldn't suffer with any problems sleeping.

I come off the booze every year now for a period of a few months. That way all of your organs come back to normal and within a short space of time, your organs will improve back to 100% normally within a few weeks. When you drink booze on a daily basis, the alcohol does interfere with the performance levels of all your organs. So obviously causes a small amount of damage. Before retiring to bed it's best not to have coffee, tea, or anything high in caffeine, even hot chocolate as that contains too much energy chemicals.

It's best to probably finish off the night with a glass of water an hour before going to bed if possible.

WISH UPON A STAR

If I could grant you a wish, what would it be? Would you opt to quit smoking and not feel any withdrawal pangs? Well I can do that for you now, just read on and finish the book and you're half way there and when you complete the simple programme devised by myself, you will end up a non-smoker in a short time of approximately six weeks, and pain free. You don't need wishes to be granted in life to be successful. It's all in your own hands. It's down to you how you lead your life. All you have to do is follow your conscience and be prepared to work and get your hands dirty metaphorically speaking. Have you noticed lately that tv. companies are using their ads to target women more to play bingo on their laptops and getting them to download their apps to download onto your mobile phone. Would you rather be given a million pounds as a gift or make the million yourself? Well i'd rather work for it because if I made a million and lost it, i'd know how to make it again. Living off adrenalin during opening hours at the Newmarket Tavern when a customer walks through the door and would end up having a drink of beer and a chat with my wife to talk about the day and what may have happened just to chill out and come down off the high adrenalin rush that normally happens every day. The thing is you never know who's going to walk through that door, also over the years I've been threathened with violence and even on one occasion with death, and at times it's not very nice to hear these threats and what to do about them, but it's part and parcel of the game, and I suppose after a lot of years one gets used to it. Some people think the pub game is an easy one but it's not, but I did love it, that's why I put up with the bad side of it because on the other side it was exciting entertaining enthralling and very rewarding. Loving your job is not like normal work it's more like a hobby and being paid for working on your hobby is just wonderful. It's not like work at all. I would suggest that all publicans would have a drink at the end of the night so they could relax enough to actually get to bed and sleep well. Sadly these days I think the writings are on the wall in the pub game and it's steadily going down the drain, because of the governments rulings on the price of a pint and also the banning of smoking in public houses and restaurants, and I can't see many of them surviving in the future, looks like we got out at the right time.

HE AINT HEAVY
(he's my brother)

When you quit smoking, you may start to worry about weight gain, well to put on more weight, you would have to eat more, so don't eat more. Smoking doesn't feed you so why would you want to eat more because you don't have a cigarette to smoke. It doesn't make sense. I knew one bloke who gave it up late in his life, he was over 60 years old and what he used to do if he started suffering withdrawal pangs was go for a walk and by the time he returned home the pangs were gone. When you stop smoking with my method, you really shoudn't suffer any withdrawal pangs as you've prepared your body in a controlled and steady way and in a slow way. Your body will be without stress because of the way you've done it. Everyone in this life should strive for fitness, and be in the right shape, and not be overweight, because you will be causing your body undue stress. As they say in life, Everything in moderation is best for all of us. Treat your body like a temple. I do feel sorry for all the poor people who are obese but the sad thing is they could fix it themselves. All they have to do is eat less and exercise more, you don't have to be Albert Einstein to work that one out, just normal and rational thinking will suffice. By using my method you are in control and by gradually reducing your intake of nicotine you are being kind and gentle to your body like a doctor would be if treating you. Also by reducing slowly you will not suffer withdrawal pangs.

YOU'VE GOT YOUR TROUBLES

A few of our customers would like to talk about their troubles and sometimes would want your advice, and as the typical landlord normally has a useful general knowledge, his advice is sought quite often on virtually any subject. He can dish out a lot of useful advice when required or even advise where to go or who to see. How many times have you heard the expression "There were exstenuating circumstances". One hears it quite a lot if you watch a lot of t. v. All it really is an excuse to get you out of a jam usually. Well what I say is this don't make excuses for not giving up smoking, just read this book and be inspired to do it or at least plan for it. There's always a reason for the smoker for not starting to quit smoking, a bad day at the office, the weathers awful and it's depressing, falling out with a friend. This decision that you make today will change the rest of your life for the better. Please do what you have to do to change your lifestyle to get the best out of it and start to plan now rather than to procrastinate.

Think of me as your guardian angel on your shoulder guiding you through your journey to stop smoking from day one right up to the end.

You might want to use me as a divine intervention, someone who's turned up just at the right time.

Isn't it time to liberate yourself and be free at last to the addiction of that demon nicotine.

Don't forget to be disciplined in your in your approach to starting to stop smoking and don't have any regrets in life.

I can't understand the celebrities of today who make staggering amounts of money over the years only to end up broke and desperate in the end. I mean how can you squander millions of pounds? I suppose studying accountancy has made me appreciate money and given me insight to investing, but also probably the way I was brought up by my parents and siblings.

The first time that I went to the dentist with my mother I was given gas and had a tooth extracted. When I was under I had a nightmare and that a train was using my teeth as railway tracks. Needless to say my dislike of dentists started that day. I was definitely fearful of ever going again. You have to overcome your fears in life if you're going to survive. We all have to face our fears and also we all have to use dentists in our lives. There was a dentist in Australia who when taking out one of my molars had a hold of my tooth with a pair of plyers and I ended up following him around the room screaming in agony. Now that was painful, I thought at one point he was going to put his foot on my chest! Thank God I never had to use him again.

EVERY DAY

The world will be a better place when you decide to take back control of your body and stop smoking and exercise more and change your diet to a better one, it will be like walking into the garden of Eden where all your favourite things are.

Maybe smokers will have to go to something like alcoholics anonymous (AA)and stand up and mention their name and add "I am an addict and I am addicted to nicotine and have been a smoker for ten years and I need help to quit smoking and become a decent human being again. Then they might have to go through a ten point plan of action to eventually come off the cigs. Being addicted to anything is bad for you. You need to get to the stage whereby when you make conscious decisions about what you drink in life. Make sure you don't end up addicted like an alcoholic. It's ok to drink, but drink sensibly and try not to overdo it, getting merry is a good thing and not getting drunk is good, but if you go overboard and become drunk, you then lose control and could end up in any sort of trouble. I would suggest that if you want to become drunk, make sure you start off in a good mood to begin with and don't make a habit of it, and it's probably a good idea to have a mate with you to help keep you out of trouble and get you home safe.

Over here in Spain, when the people of the village go out for a meal, often they will order a bottle of red wine and a bottle of water to drink one after the other and they end up sober after the meal instead of being tipsy. They never seem to get drunk and nearly always seem to be in a good mood and in good spirits. Also the children of the parents are encouraged to drink when they reach sixteen and have a drink of the red wine with a meal. A watchful eye is kept on the teenager either by the parent or the grandparent. One has to admire the way Spanish children are brought up mainly by the grandparents and they do deal out their fair share of discipline when required mixed with a lot of love and affection. I believe that's why most Spanish people have a wonderful disposition in life and are very relaxed and tranquil. Every day that you spend here on the planet is wasted if you are still smoking cigarettes. Don't waste another one, go and make a difference and make a name for yourself.

SMOKE GETS IN YOUR EYES

It's over for the poor smoker in this new world of ours. The establishments are all going against him for not being sociable and being smoke free. Nobody likes the smoker now except another smoker, but the smokers of this world are decreasing every year and eventually there will be no smokers left on the planet, so it sounds like a good idea not to be left on the shelf sad and lonely. Even the doctors of this world are saying for the future don't get ill because everything is going against the smoker and there are less doctors and nurses working in hospitals today. In the future some hospitals will refuse entry for any smokers; it's the way the world is changing. It's time to make a big decision, do you want to remain a smoker and eventually be the only smoker left on the planet when all your friends have already given up or do you want to change your lifestyle now, and keep all your friends you've had most of your life, but who have now become non-smokers. No, I don't think so because I wouldn't stay a smoker if that was to happen to me. What is left for the poor smoker to light up and enjoy that cigarette, hardly anything. First there was hospitals, cinemas, theatres, restaurants, and now pubs. Next it will be cars following in the wake of taxi's especially when children are in the car with their parents. Legislation is already afoot with the government.

Have you ever watched a t.v.programme named Nothing to declare? You wouldn't believe what people will do to get cheap cigarettes into the country, and all because they're smokers, one smoker tried to smuggle in the equivalent of forty five thousand pounds worth of cigarettes on one journey but was sniffed out by a sniffer dog and checked out by customs officers who after finding this large haul confiscated the lot. Sometimes people who know what the regulatory amounts are, normally 200 cigarettes which is normally one carton that are allowable into the country, and those same people try to cheat the system and end up with no cigarettes at all because all those cigarettes that are confiscated are incinerated. You wouldn't have to do silly things like that if you didn't smoke, so wise up now. You don't need to smoke so take control now and sort out your life. Think of a new world without having to smoke, it's unthinkable and unbelievable but the rewards are quite wonderful, no more out of breath after a walk but felling fitter than ever before. You will be able to exercise more often.

TOBACCO ROAD

To quit smoking one must understand why we are smoking in the first place is because we are addicted to nicotine which is found in tobacco which of course is found in cigarettes that we smoke. Now I'm not going to insult your intelligence, but try coming off the cigarettes without any preparation and you will receive a rude shock to the system and awakening and that is you will feel in a state of panic very quickly if you are a smoker and not had a cigarette for a while, i.e., maybe an hour or a half an hour, your body starts to go into stress mode and if not fed with a fix of nicotine which is obviously found in the proverbial cigarette, you will feel the pangs of an withdrawal symptom, and also because you will know they are very uncomfortable and is basically eating away at your stomach. That's why you are smoking today, it's not because you are enjoying it, it's because you need it! It's because you are addicted, If there was an alternative to smoking cigarettes and you actually enjoyed it, I'll bet you would change the habit tomorrow if you could, but the sad thing is there is no alternative to this dirty habit, so it's best to stop once and for all and not use any other substitute as it will only prolong the agony. I noticed on the sky news today that England is suffering badly with a fog thick with sand and grit from the Sahara desert in Africa.

Apparently the amount of people being taken to A&E has increased by over 15% as a result of the problem and the people are struggling to breathe properly. One of the main reasons for this is that most of them will more than likely smoke cigarettes and suffer with poorly chests. Don't put off the inevitable and postpone the day you'll quit and put into motion now a plan of action, also don't procrastinate any longer because global warming is not going away any day soon. The authorities are saying that global warming is here to stay and the United Kingdom is still going to struggle with severe weather conditions including flooding especially in the south of England where it flooded badly around Christmas 2013 and nearly ruined hundreds of acres of farmers land, not to mention the houses and cars. The government have only announced now that they are going to be dredging the rivers in the south so it doesn't happen again. So everything is going against the poor smoker who can't stop smoking .Oh what a shame because the smoker is not going to be able to improve his breathing because he's already choking himself to death, by continuing to smoke the ghastly cigarettes.

GET BACK

An addiction is anything we do to avoid hearing the messages that the body and soul are trying to send us. The Beatle song get back suggests that we want to get back to where we belong before we started smoking. It was useful being a humanologist and also helped me learning a bit of psychology, also to help me in my job I had to be relaxed, and that's one of the key factors. When you're a nobody and the only way to be anybody is to be somebody else, yes yourself.

My wife Linda used to smoke forty cigarettes a day, two packets of Winston here in Spain. I was smoking roll-ups at the time about ten a day so after we discussed the idea of stopping smoking, I decided on a plan of action. The first thing I did was change back to the regular taylor made cigarettes. What I did was come up with a plan a combination of all the different ways I'd given up in the past and came up with a three pronged attack. As I've discussed before is the self-hypnosis, writing a letter to yourself and signing it and reading it to yourself for basically the next six weeks. The next thing to do is if you're a forty a day smoker, the first thing you do is reduce down to twenty within a fortnight. You can set yourself targets like drop two cigs the first day and one the following day then two on the third day and so on to reach the figure of twenty a day. At least you've started so carry on now and in the third week you can drop down to ten a day by using the same method, ie, drop two a day the first day and one on the third day and set yourself the target of smoking ten per day. Once you have reached this target you are going to love the next stage. This is how it works;In your fourth week you can smoke ten cigarettes per day for three days and then reduce down to nine cigarettes per day for another three days, then from there on, I think you can see where this is going. You then keep on reducing and smoking the target set for three days at a time, until you reach smoking down to three a day, now when you reach this target You can smoke the three cigarettes for the next three days and then that's it you have reached your target and I can promise you that you won't need a cigarette again, you'll be fed up bothering with a cigarette again. So now you can get on with your life and enjoy it in a better way. You can be very proud of yourself. Well done. Bueno Hecho!! We didn't bother with two and then one cigarette because we didn't need them!

www.ingramcontent.com/pod-product-compliance
Lightning Source LLC
Chambersburg PA
CBHW032028290526
45786CB00011B/1126